NANNIES, HOUSEKEEPERS, AND CAREGIVERS

A Practical Guide to Finding Help at Home

JAYNE ANN WESTER-SMITH

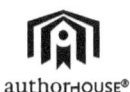

authorHOUSE®

AuthorHouse™
1663 Liberty Drive, Suite 200
Bloomington, IN 47403
www.authorhouse.com
Phone: 1-800-839-8640

First published by AuthorHouse 3/20/2008

ISBN: 978-1-4343-7338-0 (sc)

Printed in the United States of America
Bloomington, Indiana

This book is printed on acid-free paper.

Illustrations by Jayme Flythe

For further information about caregiving services send your e-mail to:
HIRING A CAREGIVER.COM

This book is dedicated to my parents,
whom I miss so much.

Special thanks:

To my sister from roller-skating to writing this book.
Thank you for always being there.

To my aunt, Elnora Johnson, for providing me
with valuable insight on caregiving.

To Nanny Care Placement Agency, San
Jacinto, California, for their support.

Table of Contents

Introduction

Families on the go, single parents, dual career families, and members of the "sandwich generation" all need help as they try to take the best care possible of their homes and of those they love. From watching over a newborn to assisting an elderly parent, at some point, almost everyone will need help around the house. This book is written for the many people who need caregivers but don't know how to conduct the search.

Opening your home to a helper can be a wonderful, rewarding experience for everyone involved, but the process takes time, and this guide can save you both time and trouble. Written by an agency owner, this is a simple and direct "how to" book that will answer some of the most common questions that people ask when seeking and hiring a caregiver in the home.

I graduated from the State University of New York College at Brockport in 1983 with a Bachelor of Science Degree in Communications. Shortly thereafter I landed a junior executive position in one of the country's leading advertising firms in Chicago. After working in corporate America for a few years, I returned to New York in the late-eighties to care for an elderly parent. I started a cleaning business that would enable me to work from home, and I began to receive numerous requests for nannies and babysitters.

1

Recognizing that there was a high demand for caregivers and no referral-placement agencies in the area, I branched out and started a referral placement agency for people who were seeking nannies, housekeepers, companions, and baby nurses. My business had been in existence for almost twenty years, averaging about 100 to 150 placements per year, some of whom were for repeat clients. After twenty years of matching caregivers and families, I learned a lot about both the client's and the caregiver's needs, and the most common concerns of both. Moreover, I learned how to foster a harmonious client-caregiver relationship. I would like to share my successful experience with others.

Today it is usual for both a wife and husband to work, leaving the care of their children to a nanny/housekeeper. We live in a time when divorce rates are skyrocketing, leaving single parents in need of childcare. Further, many of the parents of the baby-boomers need companions or home health care aides. Over the last few years, many people have called me who are bewildered about how to begin to secure the caregiving services they so desperately need.

This book is written as a simple guide to answer some of the most commonly asked questions by those who are searching for caregivers/housekeepers. It is designed to help you find a caregiver that fits your family's needs. In the following pages, ten types of caregivers are discussed. Pages are provided for you to record your specific questions and caregiving needs.

It is a big step to invite someone to work in your home. I hope the information here can guide you through the process step by step and offer your practical assistance to make the client-caregiver relationship work well. After reading this book, you will have enough knowledge to hire a caregiver and/or housekeeper either through an agency or on your own.

I. Using an Agency

A. The Benefits of Experience and Procedure

When families look for someone to help them at home, the most commonly sought caregiver* is someone who can keep the house running and care for the children, a nanny/housekeeper—most families are looking for someone who can fill both roles. But some families' needs are more specialized. Some need help to get through a temporary situation. Others may need help for years. Some families need help only one day a week; others may require five. There is also a growing need for caregivers who are able to help with elderly parents or relatives with special needs.

In seeking the right person to fill one of these positions, many people depend on word-of-mouth and are lucky enough to find a good caregiver simply on the advice of a friend. But if you have never hired a caregiver before, one of the easiest ways to gain

---

* *Although "caregiver" is associated with medical attention, in this guide, I use the term more literally—to cover someone who helps families care for their homes and loved ones. The "caregiving" I refer to here ranges from managing daily routines for healthy babies to providing assistance for bedridden seniors to finding someone who can manage a household.*

access to reliable information and applicants is through an agency. Some agencies specialize in placing nannies, companions, or housekeepers—and most agencies help place all three. This book's primary aim is to help you get the most out of working with an agency.

Before You Call

Agencies must have a state license and an office in a commercial area. Before you begin working with an agency, call the Better Business Bureau to find out if there have been any complaints about the one you are interested in. Make sure too that you have the agency's physical address.

Doing Your Homework

Once you have found an agency that you would like to do business with, your first task is to explain to the agent the type of person you are looking for. Be specific—there are a number of attributes that you should decide on before you begin the process. You may, for example, want to hire a mature, bilingual, live-in, fulltime nanny. Those are all important and specific qualifications that your agency will need to be informed about as they search for an applicant who can fulfill your requirements.

Think over and prepare your questions ahead of time—no question is silly when it comes to your loved ones, so ask away! Once you have established the type of person you would like to hire, it is the agency's task to find a match from among their pool of applicants. Most agencies have a client profile where they will store all of your information to help them select the right person to place with your family. When you have your initial interview with the agency, there are some procedural questions you should ask.

- Does the agent check all of an applicant's references?
- Do they check applicants for a criminal record?
- Do they check for a valid driver's license and for moving violations?

If they do, ask for copies of these reports. Check references on your own to make sure they are reputable.

What the Agency Does:
The Importance of Accurate Records

Most applicants looking for employment go to an agency. The agency's job is to collect the pertinent information and to make sure that information is accurate. Unless the agency specializes in au pairs, agencies interview applicants in person. An insightful agent will make the most of this initial interview. When the applicant arrives, the agent's first task is to assess appearance. Next, agents listen as applicants talk about themselves and their experiences as a caregiver. Agencies should obtain all of the applicant's degrees, licenses, and certificates to make copies of them. During the interview, agents give the job-seeker an application to complete. Besides obtaining the information on the application, watching as the applicant fills out the form allows the agent to determine whether an applicant is literate.

Agents verify the correct spelling of the name and the address on the application. Accuracy is vital, so that when the agency checks for a criminal record, the information they obtain is complete and correct. Photocopies of social security cards are also important, as are up-to-date telephone numbers. Agents should pay close attention to an applicant's driver's license number (if a number differs from the one that is on the application, the agent should ask for details. Perhaps the applicant has recently moved). Passports and visas also provide key information. Applicants come from many different countries and are in the U.S. on various types of visas. For example, an applicant may have a visiting visa, a visa to work for one year, an expired visa, etc. Some workers do not plan to return to their home country or are currently being sponsored by a family member. Some plan to stay in the United States a limited amount of time. Agents should remember to make sure that the applicant signs the bottom of the application that states that the information the applicant supplied the agency is accurate and true. All of this information is important, and a good agency will have a process in place for acquiring it.

B. Money Matters

Agency Fees and Your Caregiver's Salary

Agency fees vary from state to state. Fees may be set according to the number of hours a caregiver is working or gauged by one week's salary; sometimes the fee can be negotiated between you and the agency. Most agencies require fees paid upon placement of a nanny, but you may ask if the agency will give you a one-week trial before you actually pay the fee. With most agencies, an average fee ranges anywhere from $750-$1200 (fees for placing an au pair are much higher).

Before settling on an agency, do some comparison shopping: call at least three agencies to compare fees. Ask about the agency fee up front, and make sure the fee includes all background checks. As with any reputable business, an agency has quite a bit of overhead: agencies pay for advertising, rent, background and Department of Motor Vehicle (DMV) checks, licensing, taxes, accounting fees, bonding and insurance—all costly in today's market. Always ask what the agency fee is up front, and make sure all background checks are included.

An agency reviews information from a pool of applicants who are looking for work as nannies, housekeepers, or companions, and all of these positions have different salary ranges. Experience is one of the most important factors in determining a caregiver's salary. For example, some women have worked as nannies for two years, while others may have served in that position for ten; as with any job, experience counts. The nanny who has been in the business the longest is not going to work for the same pay as the nanny who has been working in the business only a short time. The agency will tell you what the salary structure for each applicant is. But once the agency finds people with the credentials you are looking for, it is up to you and the applicant to negotiate a reasonable and fair salary that will work well for both of you.

Remember too that the agency needs two to three weeks' notice prior to hiring. Most caregivers that sign up with an agency are looking for immediate placement, so if you want to hire someone for September 1, you should actually call the agency by the first or second week of August. You will want to have your new caregiver start a few days before you actually need her, so that you have time to teach her what your family's needs are before she begins working on her own.

Your Caregiver's Salary and Holiday Pay

Again, in determining your caregiver's salary, it is important to plan ahead and to remember that pay is required not only for day-to-day work but also for holidays, which vary from family to family. Employers need to be aware of the various religious holidays that may be important to their caregiver. Too, there are major holidays for which almost everyone has a paid day off (the major holidays are listed below, though there may be variations from household to household).

- New Year's Day
- Memorial Day
- Independence Day, July 4
- Labor Day
- Thanksgiving Day
- Christmas Day

These are major holidays for most people—here's a rule of thumb that may help: if you have a paid day off for these holidays, the caregiver should have one too. If a caregiver has been with you six months or longer and your family has planned a vacation, the caregiver should be paid for that week.

Vacations

Some families pay one week's vacation if the caregiver has been with them for six months, but most wait for one year. Employers usually prefer that the caregiver's vacation occur when the family takes their vacation. The caregiver should be paid for that week. After a year of employment, vacation time may increase, but that decision is up to the discretion of the family. As with all important issues between you and your caregiver, clear, open, considerate communication is vital.

Raises

At the end of one year, the caregiver should get a raise, even if it is a small one. Raises can be given every six months, but employers most commonly offer them once a year. Raises should start from at least ten percent of the caregiver's gross salary. Bonuses should be between one month's, or, at the very least, one week's salary.

An Alternative Way of Paying for it: Bartering

Some people may not have the income to afford paying a caregiver; one alternative is bartering. During a period of high mortgage rates and refinancing, some families desperately need some help at home but cannot pay the full rate for this help. These clients call an agency to put in a request for a caregiver who will work for a lower weekly rate; they, in exchange, give the caregiver a free place to live. This arrangement often works well for college students, single moms, and for an older or retired person.

Under this exchange, the caregiver has set hours. Monday through Friday, for example, she or he works an eight- or ten-hour a day shift. The family would pay about $200-250 a week, depending on the caregiver's duties. Any work over the agreed upon forty to fifty hours a week is considered overtime. The client should be responsible for all of the utilities. If the client does not go through an agency, he or she should advertise on college campuses, in local circulars, places of worship, and in local newspapers to look for someone willing to make this kind of arrangement.

C. Documentation and Information: Contracts, Questionnaires, and References

Pre-Contract Agreement

A pre-contract agreement safeguards an agency's investment of time and keeps expectations clear during the hiring process. Most pre-contract agreements state that you, the client, have decided to interview people through an agency. If you decide that you want to hire someone, you must contact the agency. Clients should complete and return pre-contract agreements to the agency (through email, fax, or by post) before any candidates are sent for interviews. A sample of such a pre-contract is below.

ABC AGENCY PRE-CONTRACT AGREEMENT

_____Jane Doe_____ has decided to interview potential nanny/ housekeepers through ABC Agency. If she decides to hire a candidate through our agency, Ms. Doe has been informed that the agency fee of __$750.00__ is due upon placement of the nanny/housekeeper for which a contract will follow.

__Jane Doe_____   _____
Customer Signature   Agent Signature

Contracts

Pre-contract agreements simply state that if you are interested in interviewing a caregiver through an agency that you are obligated to pay the agency fee if you hire a caregiver. The contract, however, contains much more detailed information. *Make sure you read your contracts carefully!* Confirm that your contract states what each party's duties are and what kind of guarantee the client has. A ninety-day guarantee is common with most agencies.

Your contract should specify the caregiver's duties and what salary you are paying each week. If you should ever need to replace the nanny, you need to know that your replacement is comparable to the caregiver whom you originally hired and that the contract stays the same.

This sample contract below outlines a basic agreement, letting both parties know that the placement of a caregiver has been accomplished and that this instrument is both your receipt and your guarantee. This contract requires the client's name (this should be printed) and offers space to list specific duties and/or care for family members. The contract:

1. Explains that you, the client, will owe the agency money if you accept a caregiver.

2. Explains what the fee is. The fee varies according to whether you are looking for a part- or fulltime placement; the contract is valid only if the fee is paid in full to the agency.

3. Explains the guarantee; in other words, if, within the specified period, the caregiver does not work out—through the client's decision or the caregiver's—a replacement must be made.

How quickly the agency can find a replacement varies with the agency. Most agencies will replace within the first few weeks, guaranteeing to supply referrals for jobseekers who fulfill the original requirements. If, for example, the original placement was a nanny/housekeeper with a valid driver's license, then the replacement must satisfy those same requirements.

4. Most agencies are "referral agencies"; that is, they refer caregivers to you. The agency is not the employer, and once you, the client, hire the caregiver, the caregiver becomes your employee. The referral agency is not liable or responsible for loss or damaged items in your home.

5. The last paragraph states that once the client has signed this contract, she or he is obligated to pay the agency fee; if the client does not pay the fee and the agency has to use a collection agency, whatever costs that the agency incurs become the responsibility of the client, as do any court or attorney fees.

The client must date, sign, and mail the original contract, along with the agency fee, to the agency upon hiring a caregiver. Note that the caregiver should not officially begin work until the agency receives its fee. If you do not understand your contract, hire an attorney and have him or her explain it to you. *Never sign a document if you are unsure about what its content means.*

NAME OF AGENCY
Address
Phone number

LIVE IN or OUT
NANNY/COMPANION/HOUSEKEEPER
AGREEMENT

I,_____(client) agree to use the services of **NAME OF AGENCY**, in the referral and placement of a domestic employee in my household. I am interested in the following:

_____

_____

_____

I understand and agree that:

1. I will owe a referral fee to **NAME OF AGENCY** only if I accept a referral for placement of a Nanny/ live-in or live-out/housekeeper/companion from **NAME OF AGENCY.**

2. **NAME OF AGENCY** fee is a flat $_____. This fee is due IMMEDIATELY upon acceptance of an employee, upon the following terms:

NAME OF AGENCY'S guarantee is only valid if: Full agency fee is paid upon placement of nanny/ live-in or live-out/housekeeper/companion.

3.   Should the employee I select leave the employment within four (4) months, whether through my decision or theirs, NAME OF AGENCY guarantees to supply referrals bearing the original requirements until a substitute is found. NO REFUNDS!

4.   NAME OF AGENCY is a referral agency only; it is not an employer or co-employer. The client will release NAME OF AGENCY from all liability or responsibility for any loss or damage resulting from the employment of a NAME OF AGENCY referral.

I understand and agree that if I accept a referral for full-time placement from NAME OF AGENCY, I will be obligated to pay the above-described referral fee. In addition, I further understand that in the event NAME OF AGENCY must seek collection of the above-described fee or any portion thereof, I shall be responsible to pay all costs of such collection, including court costs, reasonable attorney's fees and interest at the rate of 1 ½ % per month until paid.

_____   _____
Client - Date   Agent - Date

PLEASE SIGN & RETURN TO NAME OF AGENCY

Disagreements

Resolving disagreements between the client and the caregiver is one of the most important reasons that people use agencies. If there are any disagreements between the client and the caregiver and a mutual resolution cannot be found, an agent becomes the mediator, intervening to help the nanny and client resolve the differences. Most of the time it is better to have the client and caregiver try to resolve issues on their own. But if the client and caregiver simply cannot agree, the agency will work to replace the caregiver. If you decide that you want to replace your current caregiver, you should give him or her two weeks notice. If you do not feel comfortable replacing the caregiver and having her continue to stay in your home, give two weeks pay and have the caregiver leave immediately. The two-week notice is necessary to give each party ample time to prepare for the change.

D. Matchmaking: Collecting Information from Clients and Caregivers

The Importance of Complete Client Profiles

If the client wants to replace his or her employee, the agent must replace the caregiver as soon as possible. In order to insure a smooth transition, most agencies keep all of the client's information on file, so they can place—or replace—an applicant with your family. A sample client profile is below.

CLIENT PROFILE

In order to find the best match for your family, an agent needs accurate information about your home, your family, and the qualities you are looking for in a caregiver. Your answers to these questions will enable us to find an applicant best suited to your particular needs. Please type or write legibly.

NAME: _____

ADDRESS: _____

TELEPHONE: _____

      Home _____   Work _____

      Cell _____   E-mail _____

Type of caregiver you are looking for:

HOUSEKEEPER, NANNY, BABYSITTER,

BABY NURSE, COMPANION, or OTHER:

_____(please specify)

Circle one from each pair:

LIVE-IN or LIVE-OUT   FULLTIME or PART-TIME

WHAT LANGUAGE IS SPOKEN IN YOUR HOME ?_____

_____

HOW MANY CHILDREN ARE IN YOUR HOME?_____

THEIR AGES:_____

DO ANY OF THE CHILDREN HAVE SPECIAL NEEDS?_____

_____

IF SO, WHAT ARE THEY? _____

_____

IS ANYONE IN YOUR HOME A SMOKER?_____

DO YOU PREFER A SMOKER OR NON-SMOKER AS YOUR CAREGIVER? _____

DO YOU HAVE ANY PETS? If so, what kind? _____

_____

WHAT ARE YOUR FAMILY'S HOBBIES?_____

_____

DOES THE FAMILY TRAVEL?_____

_____

WHAT ARE THE CHILDREN'S SPECIAL LIKES AND DISLIKES?_____

_____

_____

DO YOU NEED SOMEONE WHO CAN SWIM? _____

DO YOU NEED SOMEONE WHO CAN DRIVE? _____

HOW LONG WILL YOU NEED THE CAREGIVER?_____

_____

HAVE YOU EVER HIRED A CAREGIVER BEFORE?_____

_____

IF SO, HOW LONG WAS S/HE WITH YOU?_____

_____

WHY DID THE PREVIOUS CAREGIVER LEAVE?_____

_____

WHAT IS YOUR MARITAL STATUS?_____

_____

IS EITHER PARENT A "STAY AT HOME" PARENT?_____

_____

WHAT SALARY RANGE ARE YOU PREPARED TO PAY? ____

_____

ADDITIONAL COMMENTS:_____

_____

_____

CUSTOMER SIGNATURE_____

Filling out the Client Profile: Why Agencies Need Information about Your Family

- An agency needs the client's **proper name and address** for identification and correspondence purposes.

- **Desired position:** It is important to pair a caregiver with someone looking for that caregiver's specific and desired position.

- **"Live-in or Live-out" and "fulltime or part-time"** are crucial determinants in helping the agency narrow its search to applicants willing to work those hours.

- **Language:** some families speak languages other than English. Other families may speak English as their primary language, but want someone who speaks another language, so that their children can become bilingual.

- **Number of children:** will help determine salary and help the agent find a good match.

- **Age range:** caregivers often prefer working with a certain age group; for example, some people do not want to care for a child who is not potty trained.

- **Smoker/Non-smoker:** some families prefer a non-smoker. Others may be willing to accept either.

- **Special needs:** it is important to explain to an agency if your child has any special needs. Some caregivers are equipped to care for children who have learning, speech, and physical disabilities, but not all caregivers are. Parents should not withhold information about a child's disabilities, because the child will suffer if the caregiver does not have the educational background or experience to care for that child. Accurate information at the very beginning of this process will save everyone time and inconvenience.

- **Hobbies:** allows the agency to find a caregiver who has similar interests.

- **Pets:** this information tells the agent to limit applicants to those who are neither allergic to nor afraid of animals.

- Since the children will be spending a lot of time with the caregiver, information on their **likes and dislikes** is important; such information helps the caregiver have the right information in the beginning to help her build a solid relationship with the child(ren).

- **Travel:** some caregivers have restricted visas, so caregivers need to know if clients will require them to travel. Clients need to know if the caregiver's visa allows them to travel outside of the country. Many agencies have temporary nannies on file who can be employed to travel with the family on vacations.

- **Length of time** you need a caregiver will determine whether you should hire a short- or long-term caregiver.

- **Swimmer or driver:** many families have pools or club memberships and want nannies who can swim with the children. Too, nannies shop, pick up dry cleaning, and take children to extracurricular events. Families must also find out if the caregiver has a valid driver's license.

- The agency needs to know **if you have hired before** and if you encountered problems. When it comes to finding the right person to care for your loved ones, no questions are off limits. If a caregiver has left your employ, tell the agency when she left and why. If she did not get along with the person she was caring for, explain that on the profile.

- **Marital status:** important information for the caregiver. If, for example, the parents are divorced, there may be custodial provisions that constitute days of visitation for the parent not living in the household. The caregiver must be aware of the schedules mutually agreed upon between the parents.

- Many caregivers prefer to work for a family in which there is no **"stay at home" parent**, because they feel parents will look over their shoulders, making it harder to establish authority with the children (this is a valid fear—parents hiring a caregiver often need to step into the background, especially in the beginning, to allow the caregiver to establish her authority and perform her duties).

- **Salary range:** since salaries differ according to the caregiver's experience, the agents needs to know how much the client plans to spend.

- **Additional comments:** this open-ended space for questions or comments may provide the agency with valuable information. It is important to an agent to address every comment; every answer is important in placing the right caregiver.

The Caregiver: Obtaining Information about and from the Applicant

In addition to the public agencies described in previous pages, many people also use private agencies, which are often run by retired police officers or detectives. At such an agency, a search for information on an applicant can cost anywhere from $20 to $100. If the caregiver does not have a social security number or green card, clients *must* receive a copy of the applicant's visa. The visa is often the only valid piece of identification the caregiver will have.

Gathering Information from the Caregiver: The Applicant's Profile

- **Do you have health insurance?** Some families will give employees health insurance; when hiring an au pair, health insurance is mandatory!

- **Do you have any allergies?** It's good to know what the caregivers are allergic to, so you can prevent situations that might result in a serious or even life-threatening reaction.

- **Are you afraid of pets?** Some people simply don't like to be around animals. Many people suffer from allergies, which can include pet hair and pet dander.

- **Can you travel outside the United States?** Some families that travel extensively need to know that the person has no restrictions on traveling.

- **Do you smoke?** Families may hire a smoker if she says that she would not smoke in the home or around the children. Most families, however, do not want a smoker.

- **Do you have problems caring for the elderly or physically challenged?** Giving such care requires that an applicant have previous experience, be a self-starter, and have an encouraging attitude. An agency must ask if the caregiver has a problem with a position like this because agents do not want to place a caregiver in a position in which they are not comfortable.

- Stating the **preferred age of children** with whom you like to work is very important. Some caregivers have cared only for toddlers and do not know how to take care of a newborn properly.

- **Do you swim?** If a family has a swimming pool, the may be looking for a caregiver who knows how to swim, so their children can enjoy the pool when they are not home.

- **Can you do housekeeping?** Some people want to fill a position that requires no housework;

however, most live-ins do it all! Most families
are looking for someone who can do both.

- **Can you cook?** Caregivers come from all over the world
  and many are excellent cooks, a skill highly valued by
  most families. Most families, however, are looking for
  only basic meal preparation (for example, making salad,
  baking a chicken, or putting together simple dishes).

- **What is your country of origin?** It is important for
  families to know where their perspective caregiver comes
  from. Families need to understand that if they hire someone
  from another culture that it important to make him or her
  welcome in the new home—and that what will make the
  caregiver feel welcome may be different in various cultures.

- **What language is spoken in your home?** Many families
  want their children to be bilingual; speaking another
  language is usually attractive to the prospective family.

- **Have you ever been arrested?** Agents and clients hope
  the prospective caregiver is honest in answering this
  question. Occasionally, an applicant thinks that the agency
  is not going to check, but most people know that it is wise
  to answer honestly. If the person has been arrested, it is
  up to the family to decide whether they want to interview
  them. The agency will supply all of the paperwork.

The Agent's Responsibilities
—the agency must ensure that:

- the applicant's driver's license is valid and that the picture is the person you are interviewing;

- the caregiver has at least a high school education or a GED.

Special circumstances
you may encounter:

1. Caregivers who are not citizens:

If the caregiver is not a citizen, many families will sponsor them into the United States. The caregiver's country of origin is a major factor in determining how long it will take to obtain residency or work authorization. A visa can take from fifteen months to ten years. When using the Sponsorship Program, clients should consult an attorney whose expertise lies in the legalities of sponsorship.

2. Married with Children

Some clients feel that if the caregiver is married, she may have limited hours in which to work, so they prefer someone who is not married or who is beyond child bearing age. Most people also prefer caregivers who do not have children of their own. They worry that if the caregivers' children get sick, the clients will be without a nanny. Most parents look for single people under the age of forty.

References

A few applicants come with a resume, but many don't! In order to place any caregiver, the agency must be supplied with at least one strong reference. The name, address, and phone number of the reference being used are essential. In most cases an agent will call the previous family for whom the caregiver worked.

Questions for an Applicant's Previous Employer

The agent will describe the caregiver and ask the previous employer:

- the caregiver's real name (even if a caregiver has a nickname, an agent wants to make sure that the family also knows her real name);

- what country she is from;

- her marital status;

- whether she has children;

- her legal status in this country;

- what her day-to-day duties were;

- her temperament and skill with the previous employer's children;

- her housekeeping skills;

- why she left;

- whether the family recommends her;

- whether she is personable, a self-starter, kind, nurturing; and,

- the agent will ask if the family would like to add any additional comments.

Some agencies mail out comment cards for people to fill out about their previous caregiver. Since people looking for caregivers usually want to hire one as soon as possible, it saves time simply to call. Courteous agents must ask if the previous employee would mind if their names and number were given out to potential employers who may want to hire the caregiver. (Having both home phone and cell phone numbers makes this process much easier, so agents should review the numbers with the applicant to make sure they are correct.)

Agents will find out exactly what the caregiver's duties were and the month and year they began working and the month and year they left. At least one reference should be from a place in which the applicant performed the same type of duties that she is applying for now. Clergy references are also acceptable. If the previous employer's family is moving soon, agents should get the new number, so that she or he can give the client family the new numbers.

Once all the data are compiled, the agent must wait for the results of the fingerprint and criminal background checks. As the client and potential employer, you will probably want to check the references of the applicant as well. If you call families for whom the applicant previously worked, you may want to use some of the questions above (it helps to have list of questions written down to make sure you cover everything you want to ask about). Sometimes a client may be able to find out something that the agency was unable to learn (and vice versa).

The agent will compare the applicant's data to that supplied by the client. If the agent feels comfortable with the matches, he or she calls the client about the potential candidates, and the client will contact the applicant. Some people prefer to do a phone interview before conducting an interview in person.

Families may require home help mainly in order to maintain the home and run the household, or they may need help caring for family members—from newborns to the elderly. Some families require both. In the next section, I list the definitions and duties of a variety of caregivers that you might want to employ: first, those who care primarily for children, then for the home, then for those whose role is more medical—caring for newborns and for the elderly. These positions run the gamut from those requiring little training and expense to those for which the caregiver must be educated and experienced—and who must be paid accordingly.

II. Types of Childcare Givers

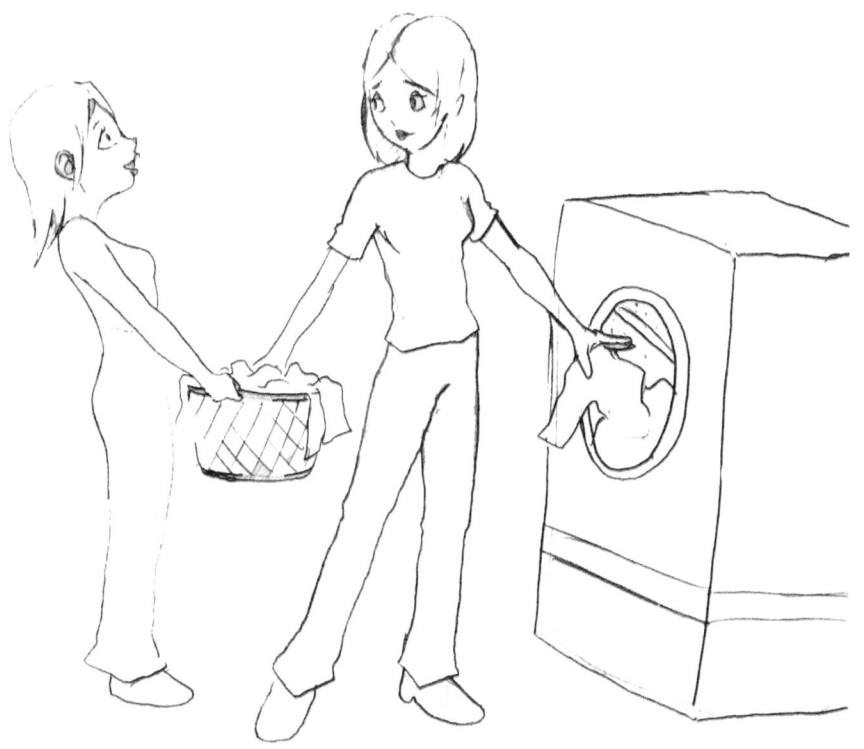

Mother's Helper

Mother's Helper

A "mother's helper" is usually an adolescent between the ages of 13-17 who helps parents with the children and light household duties. This kind of caregiver is never left alone: their job is to assist a parent with the children while the parent is at home. A mother's helper earns between $5 and $10 an hour. The usual duties of such a caregiver include:

- playing with the children;
- preparing a sandwich or giving a child a snack;
- emptying the dishwater;
- helping children tidy their bedrooms;
- sweeping the kitchen floor and vacuuming the play area.

A mother's helper should be mature and responsible enough to care for a child of any age who is at least one year old. A mother's helper is usually a neighbor or a friend who has close ties to the family. Many referral agencies have lists of mother's helper applicants, as do local places of worship.

Record Your Needs, Questions, and Important Numbers

_____

_____

_____

_____

_____

_____

_____

_____

_____

_____

_____

_____

_____

_____

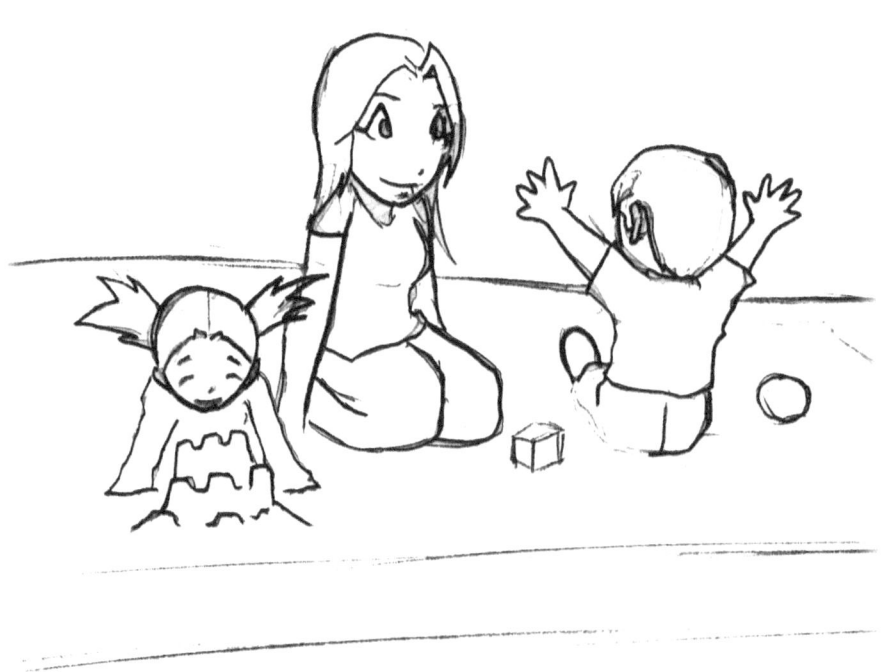

Babysitter

Babysitters

Babysitters provide childcare part-time on an "as needed" basis. They are usually teenagers (though occasionally families can find a college student or older adult who would like to earn a little cash by providing some part-time childcare). No special training is required, though many babysitters have taken a basic first aid course, and some, for instance those who are trained as lifeguards, have learned CPR.

You must know and feel comfortable that your sitter is responsible and mature enough to handle any situation that might occur with a small child. Even so, it is very important to keep important names and phone numbers posted on the refrigerator or some other easily accessible spot at all times. With teenaged sitters especially, parents must communicate rules and expectations clearly.

Babysitters should be able to play games, make arts and crafts, and read stories to the children under their care. They should also be able to prepare a light meal or a snack, supervise a child's bedtime routine, and put the child to bed. Most babysitters are very young, so their duties are limited. A babysitter should work for only about four to six hours, mostly for parents who will be away for a few hours in the evening. Babysitters normally earn between $5 and $10 an hour, depending on how many children they are caring for, how experienced they are, and how much in demand they are.

Record Your Needs, Questions, and Important Numbers

_____

_____

_____

_____

_____

_____

_____

_____

_____

_____

_____

_____

_____

_____

_____

_____

_____

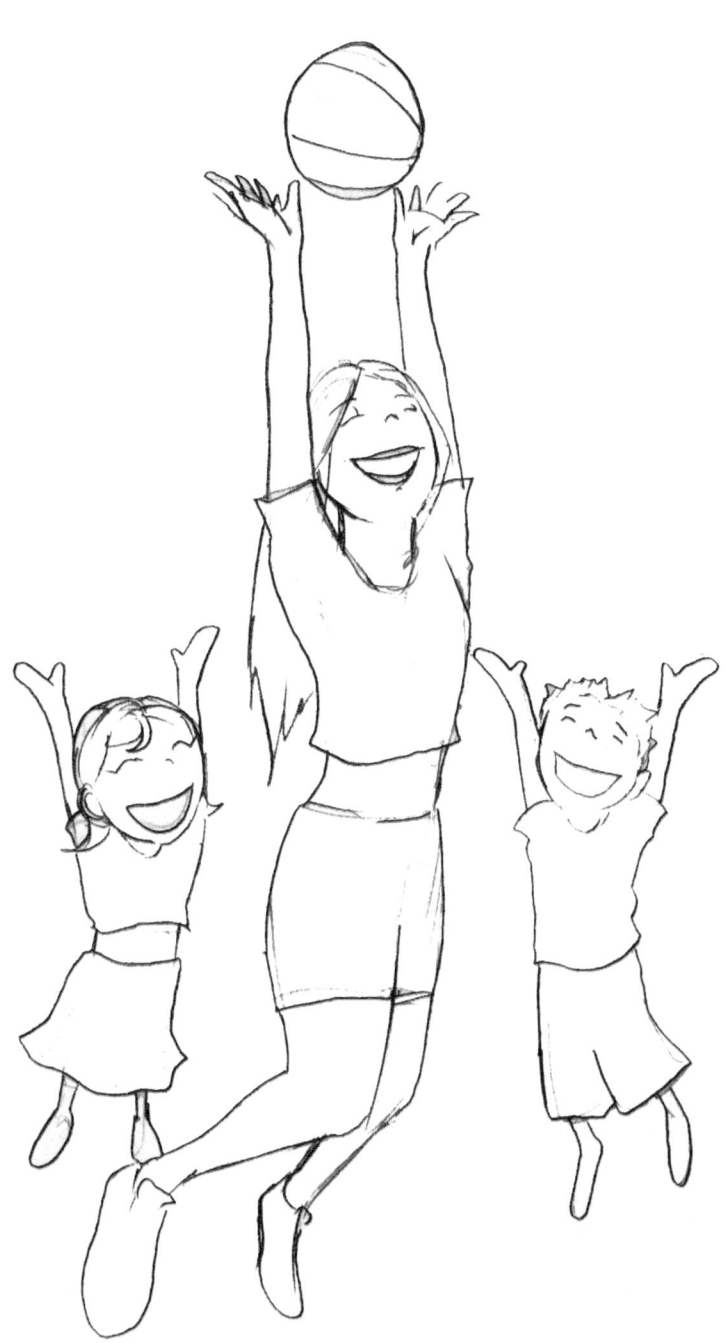

Au Pair

Au Pairs

An "au pair," is a term derived from French, which means "on par with" or "equal to"; the term describes a young woman (or, sometimes, a young man) who comes to the United States to live for a year or two. She offers her services as a child care provider in return for the chance to live with a family and perfect her English. As the term suggests, she is to be considered an equal, a member of the family, not a servant. An au pair comes to this country under a strict government-regulated program and is usually between the ages of 18-21 years old, speaks English, has no children, and is not married. Under this program, the au pair stays with a family for at least one year. Au pairs generally have student visas. Many au pairs end up being sponsored by their employers and become citizens in this country. They need an international driver's license, so they can transport children to extracurricular activities. An au pair's duties are:

1. preparing children's meals;

2. cleaning children's rooms;

3. doing light housework, associated with caring for the children, such as emptying the dishwasher in the morning;

4. doing the children's laundry;

5. helping children with homework;

6. playing with children after school; and

7. driving them to appointments.

Au pairs work eight hours per day, and their salaries range from $125-$180 per week. Au pairs normally have use of a family car on weekends and are to be treated as part of the family.

According to the U.S. State Department, au pairs provide limited childcare for a host family up to one year, and they may apply for extensions for a second year. Generally, an au pair is not to care for infants younger than three months old. The only exception is when a parent or responsible adult is at home, or if the au pair has 200 hours of documented infant care experience. Au pairs are not to be placed with a family that has a child with special needs unless they have written proof of experience, skills, or training. An au pair is limited to ten hours per day maximum—forty-five hours a week at most. Au pairs are compensated for their work according to the Fair Labor Standard Act. Participants in the au pair program must speak English and must complete at least six hours of academic credit or its equivalent at an accredited U.S. post-secondary educational institution. The family is required to pay up to $500 toward the au pair's academic course work. Since au pair programs are very popular, a great deal of information about them is readily available. A good place to begin research on this type of child care is at the State Department's website: http://exchanges.state.gov/education/jexchanges/private.htm.

Record Your Needs, Questions, and Important Numbers

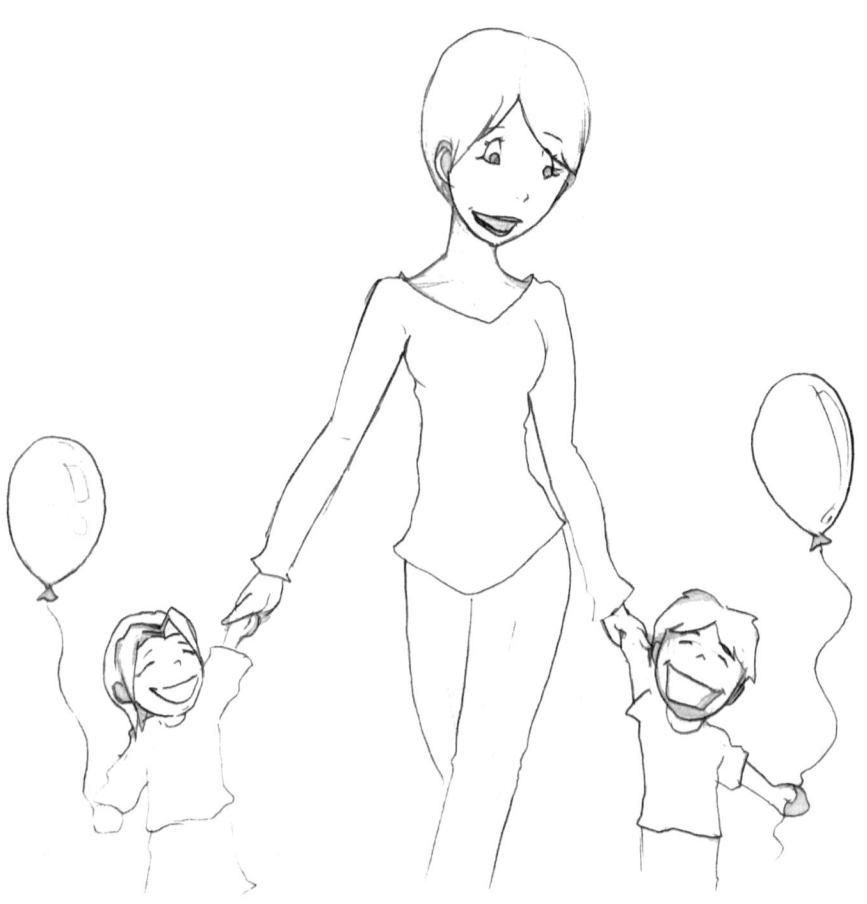

Nanny

Nannies

A nanny's job is in some ways similar to an au pair's. Nannies work similar hours—between forty and fifty hours a week. Like au pairs, a nanny's primary responsibility is for the children: they play with them, supervise homework, and take them to extracurricular activities. Nannies help children learn manners, how to behave, and they help guide children's emotional development and growth.

They may live in or live out. Nannies typically work five days a week (usually Monday through Friday or Tuesday through Saturday). Some nannies live in and work only three to four days each week. While some caregivers have childcare experience either with their own families or by caring for the children of friends, other caregivers have taken part in more formal training, such as classes in childcare and education. Nannies should be trained in first aid and CPR. Contact your nearest Red Cross organization for information regarding first aid and CPR classes.

Nannies' other duties include keeping the children's rooms clean, preparing their meals, setting up play dates, emptying the dishwasher, and mopping kitchen floors. Salaries vary by experience and educational background. The average live-in nanny earns between $400 and $700 per week. Live out nannies make anywhere from $12 to $15 per hour, depending on duties, educational background, number of children, and whether any of the children have special needs. Some nannies use their own cars, so the family pays them a weekly gas allowance, and, in some cases, reimburses them for routine maintenance, such as an oil change.

Record Your Needs, Questions, and Important Numbers

_____

_____

_____

_____

_____

_____

_____

_____

_____

_____

_____

_____

_____

_____

_____

_____

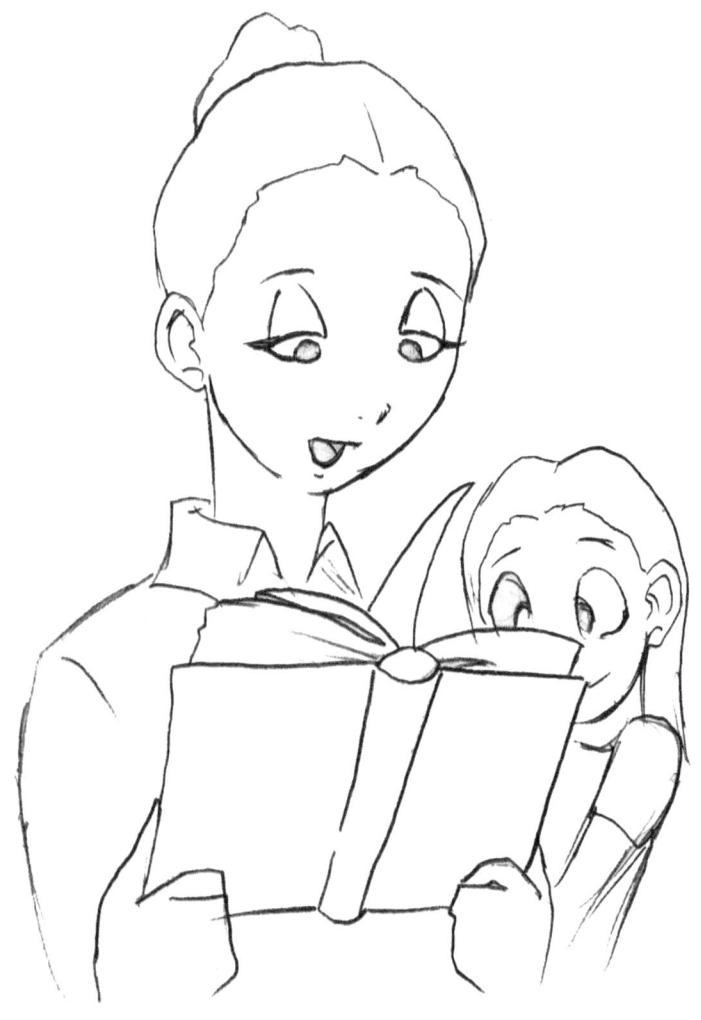

Governess

Governesses

Though we may associate this term with Victorian novels, the position of "governess" is still required by many families who want an educated caregiver who can fill two roles at once. A governess is both a nanny and an educator. She oversees the day-to-day upbringing of the children. The governess plans the children's meals and activities and directs the children on how to behave and what to wear. A governess is also trained as a home tutor. She may travel with the family abroad as a companion to the children, and, of course, must have a valid passport. A governess does not perform any household duties, but she does direct household staff on issues pertaining to the children.

A governess may live in or live out Monday through Friday or Tuesday through Saturday, putting in an eight- to ten-hour day. The pay scale is normally $1,200 to $2,000 a week, depending on the governess's level of education (for example, a governess may hold an advanced degree, perhaps even a Ph.D., in early childhood development or some other pertinent field). A governess's educational credentials are much higher than those of a nanny. In many cases, a governess is fluent in two or more languages.

Record Your Needs, Questions, and Important Numbers

_____

_____

_____

_____

_____

_____

_____

_____

_____

_____

_____

_____

_____

_____

_____

III. Caring for the Home

Suppose your need is not so much for childcare as for house care, or you need someone who can help take care of both children and the home. This section describes the duties of three types of caregivers who can help you run your home.

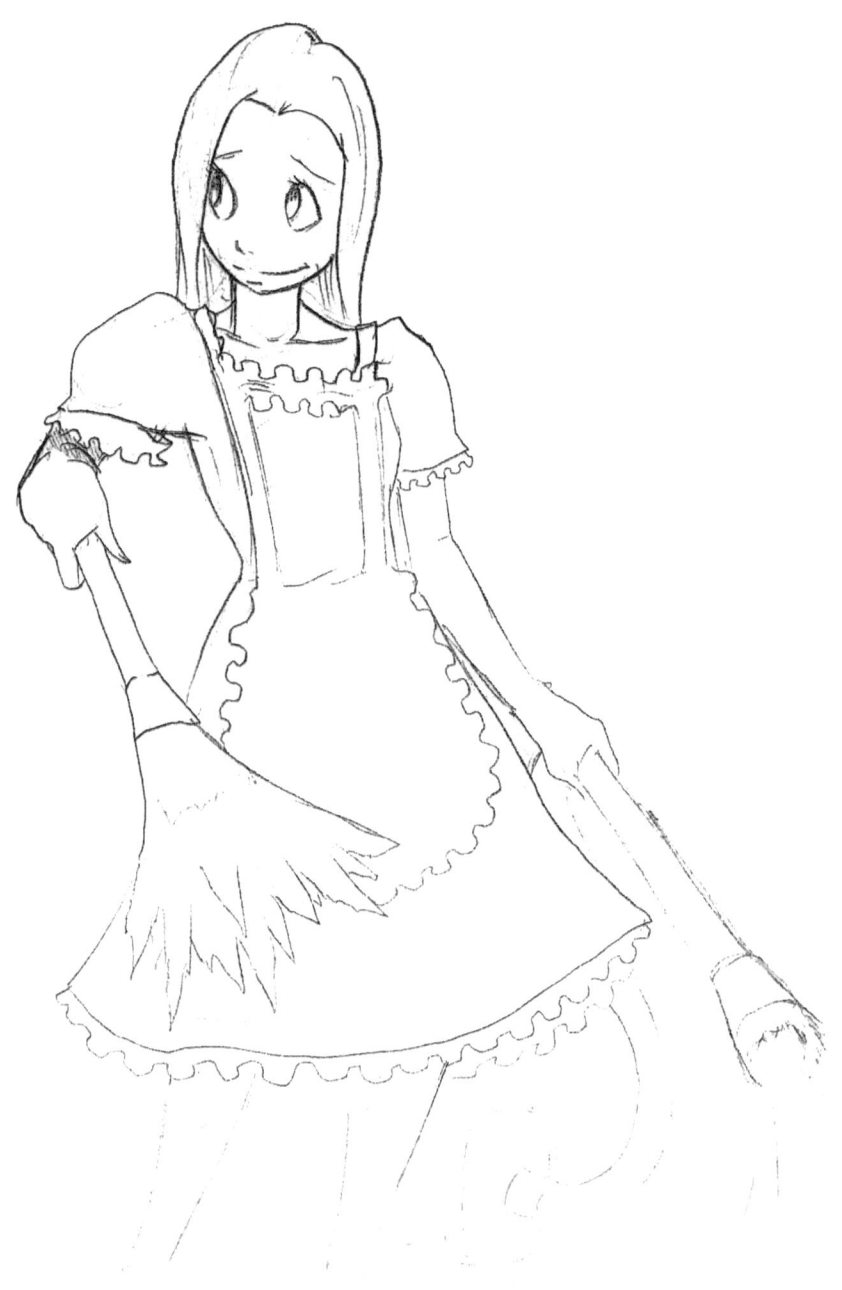

Housekeeper

Housekeepers

"Housekeeper" too is a word that may conjure visions of *Upstairs, Downstairs,* but far from being a holdover from the past, housekeepers are much in demand. Their jobs entail caring for the house, rather than the children. They may live in or live out and work full- or part-time. Housekeepers' duties vary each day, but the following are the basic housekeeping chores:

- mopping, sweeping;

- dusting;

- doing the family laundry;

- polishing furniture;

- changing linens;

- maintaining bedrooms;

- keeping kitchen appliances clean; and

- cleaning and sanitizing bathrooms.

In addition to cleaning the house, housekeepers may also be required to supervise plumbers, painters, carpet cleaners, etc. if the homeowner is not at home. Housekeepers usually work from eight to ten hours a day. A live-out housekeeper can make anywhere from $10 to $20 an hour, depending on her duties. A fulltime, live-in housekeeper earns between $400 and $600 a week.

Record Your Needs, Questions, and Important Numbers

_____

_____

_____

_____

_____

_____

_____

_____

_____

_____

_____

_____

_____

_____

_____

_____

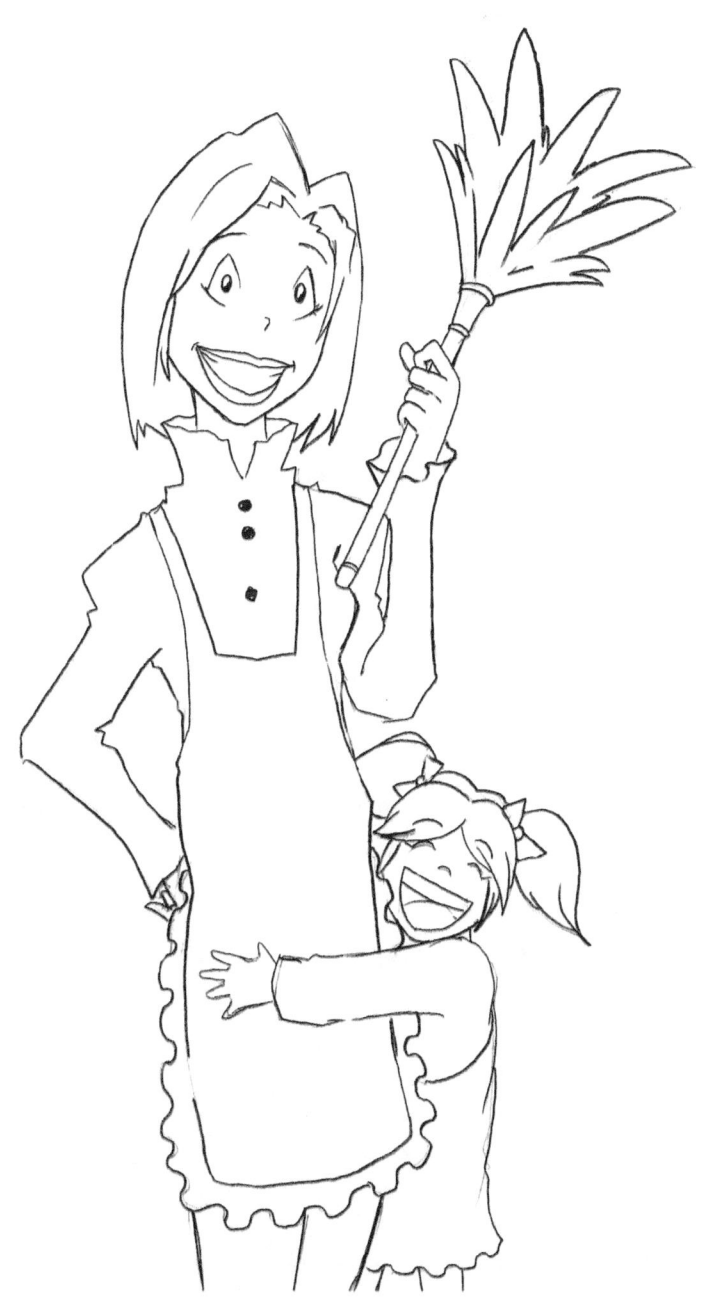

Nanny/Housekeeper

Nanny/Housekeeper

As the dual name suggests, this position requires someone willing to perform two demanding jobs simultaneously. Common wisdom says that if you have a nanny/housekeeper, you won't get both: either you have a great nanny and careless housekeeper or an inattentive nanny who keeps an immaculate house. This position entails performing the full job of a nanny—caring for the children in every capacity—and carrying out the all housekeeping duties as well. In addition, a nanny/housekeeper prepares meals for the entire family and does the family's laundry.

Nanny/housekeepers normally work Monday through Friday or Tuesday through Saturday, forty to fifty hours a week. Caregivers seeking to fill these positions should have some experience taking care of children and housekeeping in someone's home within the last year. As a live-out, a nanny will normally work for ten to fifteen dollars an hour; they generally have their own transportation.

Record Your Needs, Questions, and Important Numbers

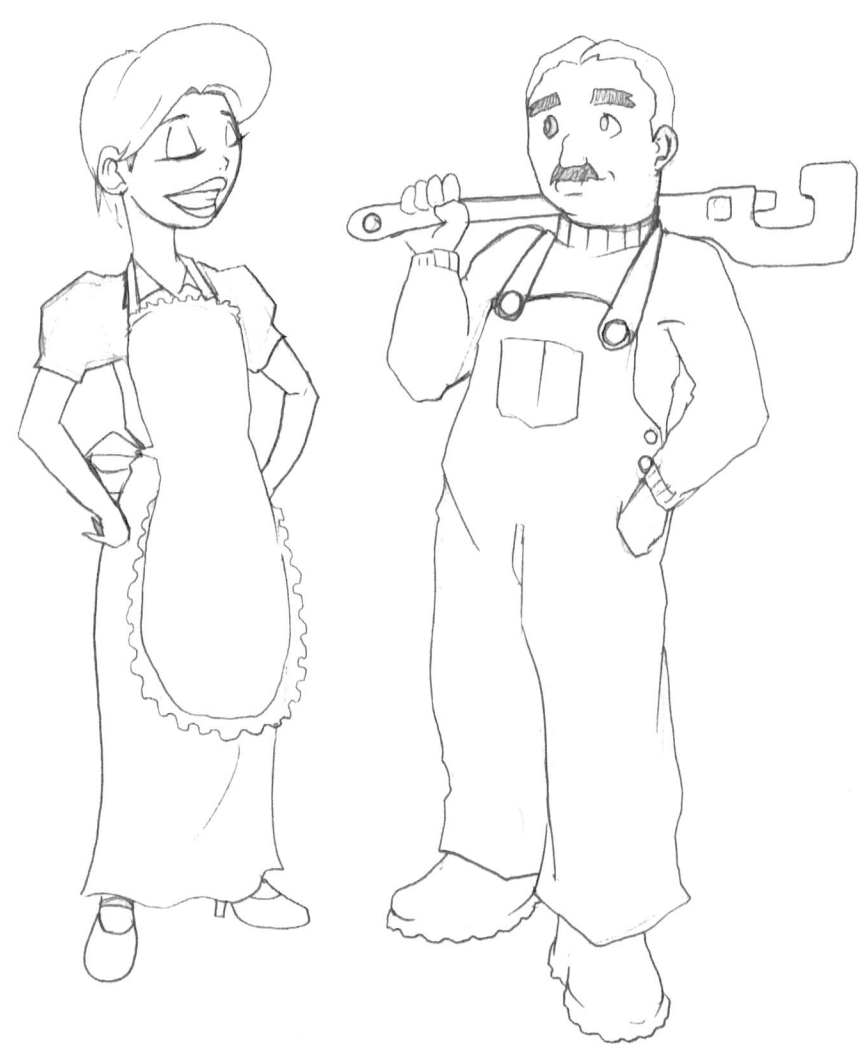

House Manager

House Manager

Even more complex than the position of nanny/housekeeper is that of house manager. House managers run the household, do or supervise the housework, and care for the children. According to *4nannies*.com (http://4nannies.com), house managers are in great demand, since so many parents work long hours. The duties of a house manager include:

- making doctors' appointments;
- taking children to extracurricular activities;
- arranging play dates;
- preparing food;
- planning parties;
- shopping for food;
- picking up dry cleaning and doing other errands;
- helping children with homework;
- changing linens;
- vacuuming and dusting;
- doing laundry;
- taking pets to the vet or groomer.

A house manager also oversees other vendors, such as plumbers, windowwashers and landscapers. Since the house manager has full responsibility for the children and the house, she must be independent—a self-starter who is able to respond to problems quickly. A house manager may receive anywhere from $100-$150 a day as a live-out. As a live-in, she (or he) may receive between $550 and $750 a week.

Record Your Needs, Questions, and Important Numbers

_____

_____

_____

_____

_____

_____

_____

_____

_____

_____

_____

_____

_____

_____

_____

_____

IV. Caring for the Vulnerable

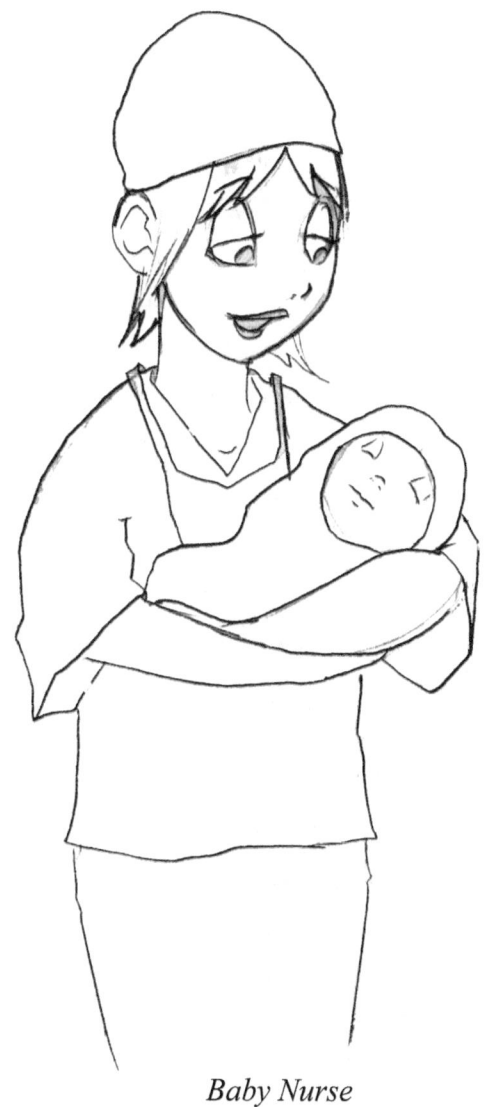

Baby Nurse

Life's beginnings and its end—maybe your needs are for care and companionship for those who are most vulnerable. Baby nurses and companions can help. Some of these positions are described in the pages that follow.

Baby Nurses

Baby nurses—doulas—help ease the early weeks of a new baby's arrival. Baby nurses usually are trained in newborn care. In many states, doulas are certified baby nurses, so they are certified in CPR and qualified to oversee the general well-being of an infant. A baby nurse has a temporary assignment with a family, which can range from two to twelve weeks. The length of time that the nurse stays depends, in part, on the condition of the baby; for instance, a "preemie" or a baby suffering from some kind of complication will require the longer stay. The nurse may work between ten- to twelve-hour shifts either day or night. Usually a baby nurse lives in until the assignment is completed.

A baby nurse is responsible for providing assistance to parents during the post- delivery recovery period and helping with all aspects of newborn care: feeding, bathing and changing the newborn, doing laundry, washing bottles, and helping parents schedule feedings. The baby nurse not only cares for the baby; she also teaches the new family how to take care of their newborn.

As with any other caregiver, a baby nurse should have her own room. Baby nurses earn from between $100 to $500 per day, depending on the number of hours and on the number of babies (singleton, twins, or triplets). Baby nurses are contracted for a minimum of two weeks.

Record Your Needs, Questions, and Important Numbers

Companions

Companions assist others with their day-to-day lives, and most companions are employed by those who need help caring for an elderly relative. The caregiver's salary will be determined by how much care the client needs. Depending upon the duties required, a companion's pay starts at around $400 per week. Companions work forty to fifty hours a week; they may live in or live out. The average salary for a companion usually ranges from ten to fifteen dollars an hour for a live out. A live-in is paid $400-$600 a week, depending on the level of care required by the client. A companion will:

- do some light housekeeping (emptying the dishwasher, sweeping the kitchen floor, wiping down counter tops, washing some laundry);
- shop for food with the client;
- take the client to doctors' appointments
- take the client for walks or to see a movie;
- travel with the client;
- assist in helping the client take medications (a companion *never* administers meds);
- assist in preparing meals;
- other day-to-day duties that may arise.

Record Your Needs, Questions, and Important Numbers

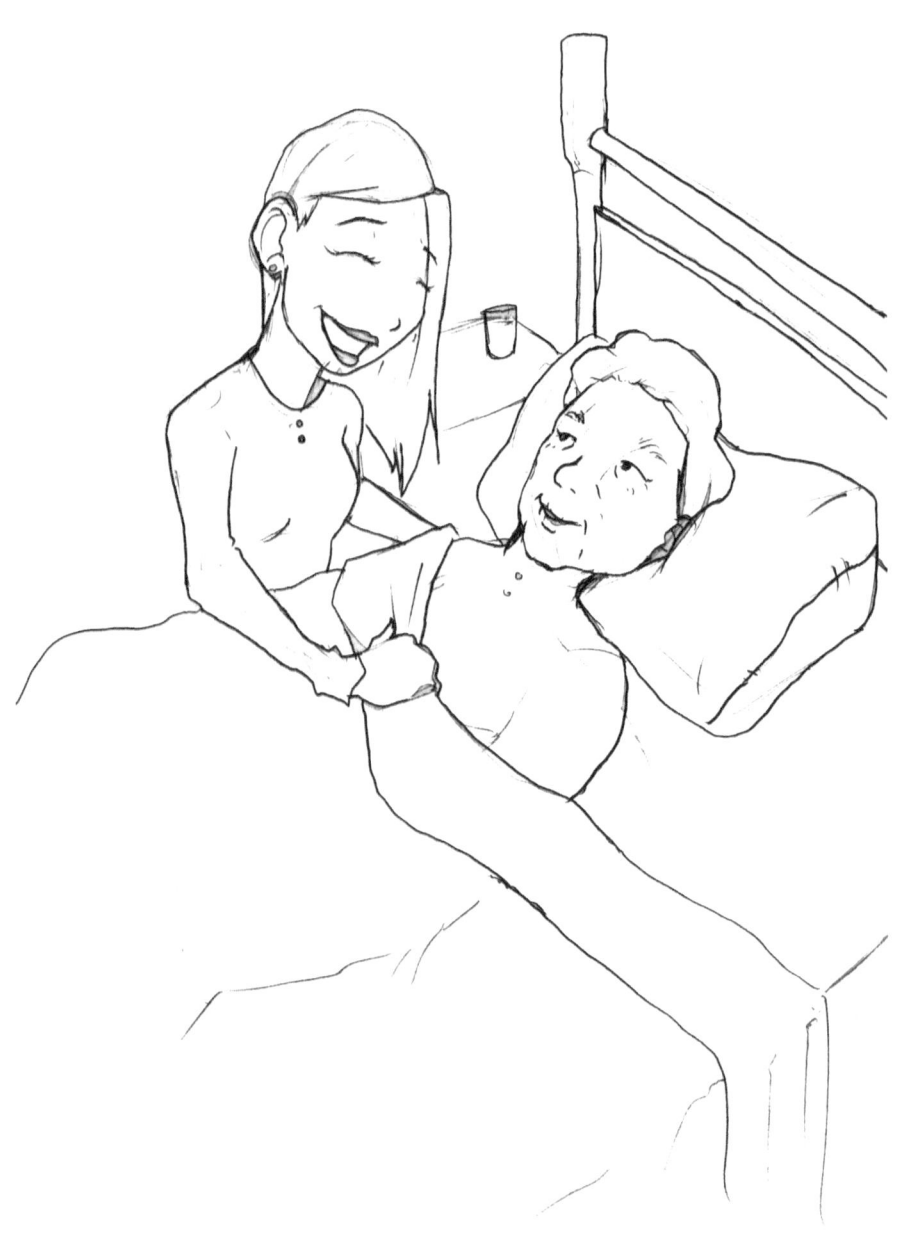

Certified Nurse's Aid

CNA (Certified Nurse's Aide)

CNAs have specialized knowledge about geriatrics and disabled people. They must be in good mental and physical health themselves. This position requires someone who is a self-starter and able to multitask. A CNA must be willing to assist with the following:

- changing linens;
- housekeeping;
- lifting and turning;
- preparing meals;
- doing laundry;
- assisting in administering meds;
- changing bedpans;
- bathing;
- feeding;
- shopping for food;
- taking patients to doctors' appointments.

Depending on the case, a CNA may be required to do all the duties listed above or, perhaps, only a few. Patience and being able to take directions from family members are crucial. CNAs earn from ten to twenty dollars an hour, depending on the severity of the patient's condition. Like all caregivers, CNAs work Monday through Friday or Tuesday through Saturday and have two days off. Very rarely do they work seven days a week. Many clients need help seven days a week, so these clients often hire a weekend caregiver as well.

Record Your Needs, Questions, and Important Numbers

_____

_____

_____

_____

_____

_____

_____

_____

_____

_____

_____

_____

_____

_____

_____

V. Less Common Situations Requiring Childcare

Child Mediators

In rare cases, a family requires the services of a childcare mediator. These are women or men who have education and training in child development. In some states, mediators are appointed through the courts to supervise visits between a parent and child. Consider the following scenario: a mother accuses the father of abusing or molesting their five-year-old daughter. The parents divorce, and the daughter lives with the mother and her new husband. In such a case, the courts might rule that the child have temporary supervised visits in a public place when she sees her father. The childcare mediator's job is to observe the interaction between father and daughter for as long as these supervised visits are recommended by the court. Mediators earn between ten and twelve dollars an hour and are paid by the parents.

Temporary Sitters

Childcare assignments of fewer than six months are considered short term assignments. Other short term assignments may be for parents who work rotating shifts for a few months or who need a babysitter on call to provide care on an as needed basis for special engagements. For arrangements like these, families call the agency and pay a flat fee (usually about $500), and the agency will guarantee a sitter once a month for twelve months or for a maximum of twelve times. The family must give at least one week's notice. There are also "temp sitters" who travel out of the country with families because their nannies don't have valid visas. This may cost a family about $300 through an agency. The family pays the caregiver directly.

Services for the Elderly and Special Needs Children

There are also facilities in many areas that will take a child that has special needs and care for the child temporarily; this occurs most often when families must go away for a while, and the child needs extensive care. Of course, this could also occur with an elderly relative; some nursing homes provide this same service.

Many senior centers and nursing homes also provide daytime care; sometimes it is less expensive to go through a senior center or nursing home for daycare or periodic overnight care. Parents of children who have special needs can usually find care provided by the government, if they consult with social services, since that level of care is usually federally funded.

Record Your Needs, Questions, and Important Numbers

_____

_____

_____

_____

_____

_____

_____

_____

_____

_____

_____

_____

_____

_____

VI. Hiring without an Agency: Finding Someone on Your Own

The internet, pennysaver, newspaper, or local places of worship all offer ways to find a caregiver on your own. You could place an advertisement or look for those that applicants have placed.

Advertising

If you place an ad for a caregiver, it should look something like this:

Nanny/Housekeeper Needed

Family of four seeks fulltime nanny/housekeeper

to live in Monday-Friday.

Children: 8 and 12 years old. Two cats.

Must have valid driver's license and speak English.

Call 216-555-5555

This information will help the potential nanny know right away if this is a position she would like to apply for. A nanny wants to know how many children are in the household and their ages, since some have a preference when it comes to the ages of children. You need to state that the applicant must have a valid driver's license, because some people are under the assumption that a driver's permit is sufficient. (When you meet the applicant, ask to see the driver's license and copy down the license numbers and expiration date). If you have pets, you need to include that information in your ad, since many people are allergic to or fearful of animals. Including such key information is important to getting off to the right start with an applicant who may become part of your household.

Conducting Your Own Criminal Search

You can give yourself additional reassurance about an applicant by doing your own search, as long as you have the correct name—the correct *spelling* of the name is imperative—date of birth and social security number. With this information, a search company can conduct a criminal search and get back to you with the following:

Jane Doe, DOB 2/2/58,
has no criminal activity as of 12/12/07.

If you end up using an agency, make sure to get a copy of the criminal search report and any information they have obtained from the Department of Motor Vehicles—after all, you have paid for it! You are entitled to any information that pertains to the caregiver you are hiring.

A search done with the DMV will let you know if the applicant has ever been ticketed for serious driving offenses, such as drunken driving. The report will state:

Jane Doe, DOB 2/2/58, received a charge
of DWI on October 5, 2005.
New York State license is suspended. No
further information provided.

Make sure that you have all of this information before the caregiver begins working in your home. Search companies are listed both on the web and in the yellow pages, so finding someone to conduct a search is easy.

Interviewing the Applicant

Once you are in contact with an applicant, you will want to set up an initial interview. Be sure to schedule your first meeting at a public place, such as a local diner or coffee shop. Before you meet, check to make sure the applicant is forthright and reputable by calling search companies and giving names and addresses of the applicant's references to make sure that they are actually at that number and address. Important numbers that will aid you in your search include the applicant's social security number and the numbers on file at the Department of Motor Vehicles (see section above). Ask for a picture ID, and make sure your background checks are thorough. Verify that the applicant is not a pedophile. Find out the last three places the applicant has lived within the last eight years.

Once you have completed your search and feel comfortable that the applicant is someone you can trust, ask her to come to your home to meet your family. Have a list of questions ready to ask the applicant. (A sample list is included at the end of this section. The "applicant's profile" in the "Matchmaking" section contains useful questions too.) Take notes during the interview. This will help you discuss the answers with the family after she leaves. These notes will also be useful when it is time to compare answers with those of other caregivers.

While you should interview as many applicants as needed, don't overwhelm yourself with interviews. Once you have chosen two or three candidates, give them a one-week trial period to see how they work out. After that, you and your family should make a decision. Remember to let the caregiver know that there is a trial period. Once the trial is over, the decision to hire should be immediate. If you delay at that point, you might lose the chance to hire someone who is a good fit.

If you hire a caregiver who drives, make sure that she has either a valid U.S. driver's license or a valid international license. Be sure to make a copy. If the new caregiver is driving her own vehicle, make sure the car is properly registered and insured for other passengers. Caregivers who use their own cars should be reimbursed for their gas. If the nanny drives the family's vehicle, make sure the caregiver is added to your policy.

Know your finances before hiring a caregiver. Caregivers can be costly but rewarding and helpful in the long run. All salaries are negotiable between client and caregiver. Always find out what the caregiver's hourly or weekly salary was with the previous family. This will help you gauge whether or not you can afford to hire the caregiver you have interviewed. Compare the job description that you have to that of the previous employer. For instance, you may want only a nanny, while the previous employer paid for a nanny/housekeeper. The lighter load in the job you are offering would then be reflected in the salary. In most places, the average salary for a fulltime, live-in caregiver runs between $10 and $25 per hour. Unless otherwise specified, caregivers are paid weekly.

Interviewing the Applicant

Once you have figured out the avenue that you want to take in finding a nanny—using an agency or searching on your own—sit down with your spouse or a friend to discuss what type of person you are looking for. Know what your basic requirements are; for example, you might know that you want a mature woman, who is bilingual and doesn't smoke. Of course, every family is unique, but the following questions can help you come up with the areas you want to cover when you interview applicants.

- Where are you from?

- Do you have a family?

- Where do they live?

- How old are you?

- Where did you go to school?

- Where do you currently live?

- Do you have any illness we should be aware of?

- Do you smoke?

- Are you pregnant?

- Would you mind taking a physical?

- Do you know CPR?

- Do you speak any other languages?

- Is English your first language?

- What ages of children have you cared for?

- Have you ever cared for a child with special needs?

- Can you do housekeeping?

- Can you cook?

- What are some of the things you like to do?

- Do you like animals?

- Can you swim?

- Do you drive?

- Do you have any moving violation citations?

- Have you ever driven in the _____?

- Can you travel outside the United States?

- How long can you work with a family? Less than one year, one year, two years or indefinitely?

- Are you available weekends?

During this interview, explain your house rules (for example, using the phone, watching television during the day). You need to find out all you can, especially if the applicant will be caring for a newborn or a child too young to talk. The one-week trial period is invaluable in seeing how the caregiver interacts with the family.

If you decide you would rather work through an agency, call the Better Business Bureau to find out if there have been any complaints about the agencies you are considering. Detailed information about agencies is covered in the earlier portions of this book.

Other Solutions to Childcare Problems

Most states have childcare councils or childcare directories. These councils or directories provide families with many childcare options. Childcare councils provide listings of agencies, daycare centers, and individual daycare providers in their home. These lists open opportunities for families on a tight budget to get the help they need. For those who want to make sure that their children interact with other children, there are also daycare providers who care for children in their homes. Like many of the services described in earlier portions of this guide, these services are available both fulltime and part-time.

VII. After the Hire

"Someone to watch over me"

Nanny surveillance cameras, better known as "nanny cams," are very common among many families who have childcare givers. Although background and reference checks are done, many people feel a need for extra assurance when it comes to their families. Nanny surveillance cameras are used to watch caregivers, of course, but they are also popular as a way to monitor children playing in the yard.

Employers would be wise never to let anyone know if they have a surveillance camera in the home. If a caregiver knows she is under surveillance, she may quit, feeling that her employer does not trust her. Most nanny surveillance cameras are hidden in areas where no one would expect them—for example, in the bindings of books, in DVD players, clocks, and smoke detectors. Employers hide these cameras anywhere the nanny and children are together frequently. Easily available from stores and websites, nanny surveillance equipment costs start at $200.

Dos and Don'ts
Practical Tips to Create
a Friendly Atmosphere

First, the things to avoid:

<u>DON'T</u>

- stay out late during the week without letting the nanny know what you are doing. Although she may live in Monday through Friday (or seven days a week), she still requires time to herself.

- refer to your caregiver as "my girl." Most caregivers are adults; many have children or grandchildren of their own— address and refer to them respectfully.

- leave a large quantity of money or jewelry in the house. There is no use in tempting anyone: put valuables away in a safe deposit box.

- require the nanny to go straight to her bedroom when the parents come home: this practice creates a separation issue.

- require the nanny to do things that are outside of her contracted agreement (e.g., washing windows or gardening).

Some practices to adopt to keep your relationship running smoothly:

<u>DO</u>

- make the caregiver feel comfortable about telling you things about the job that she does or does not like. Keeping a line of communication open keeps a relationship healthy.

- ask the nanny if she would like to sit down with the family to eat. This fosters a harmonious atmosphere and allows the nanny and children a chance to discuss their day.

- make a list of things that you expect the nanny to do on a daily basis and keep it posted in an area she will see each day. The list might say, for example: empty the dishwasher, mop the kitchen floor, and do the laundry. Explain how often you expect these things to be done, so that there is no misunderstanding later.

- list important telephone numbers in a conspicuous place, so that everyone can find it.

- give a raise once a year. Such an act shows your appreciation and will help you hold on to a good employee. The raise should be between one week's and one month's salary.

- require your children to respect the person in charge. Of course, you should always do the same—after all, they are caring for what you prize most.

- let the nanny know what a great job she is doing.

Practical Issues:

Answers to the Ten Most Frequently Asked Questions

Q. What type of living arrangements must we provide for a live-in caregiver?

A. The caregiver must have a furnished bedroom, with cable television; it is up to you whether she shares the family bathroom or has one for her own use.

Q. How should I pay the caregiver?

A. Pay cash, unless other arrangements are made.

Q. What happens if I decide that I no longer need a caregiver and my guarantee has not expired? Can I get a refund?

A. No. You have gone into the contract understanding that you have accepted the caregiver. The agency does not refund money, but an agency will replace the caregiver.

Q. Are criminal background checks done on all caregivers?

A. No. Many caregivers are in the United States on temporary visas and do not have social security numbers. It is up to the agency to have copies of the visas on file.

Q. Must we pay for transportation?

A. Paying for transportation is up to the family.

Q. Do I have to pay for medical insurance?

A. No, caregivers must provide their own medical insurance, unless the family chooses to pay for insurance for their caregiver.

Q. How can I be sure a caregiver is not going to harm my child?

A. Criminal background and reference checks are a must. If you are still not comfortable, use a nanny camera.

Q. Must I provide the caregiver with meals?

A. Yes. If the caregiver lives in, ask what her preferences are when you shop for food. Purchase what she likes, if it is within your budget.

Q. After hiring the caregiver, how will I be sure she or he will stay?

A. Caregivers that are under a sponsorship program are likely to stay longer, because they are seeking citizenship status.

Q. Are live-ins paid more or less of a salary than live-outs?

A. Generally, live-ins are paid less than a live-outs, because they receive room and board.

Epilogue: Some Cautionary Tales from the Annals of an Agency Owner

As the former owner of an agency, I have interviewed some interesting clients and applicants. Below are a few scenarios that illustrate a variety of problems that agents, applicants, and clients can easily avoid. It takes courage, flexibility, and good humor to open one's home to someone else. It takes those same qualities to move in to another's home, ready to provide good care for a variety of needs. But the client-caregiver relationship can run smoothly if everyone involved communicates clearly, deals honestly, and infuses interactions with some good will and good humor. Below are some of the most interesting cases from my files.

Scenario 1:
Sabotaging the Caregiver

I once interviewed an applicant who had worked for a family for five years. This 32-year-old woman was part of the family. The young children adored her. She was like a much loved relative: when her mother visited from the Philippines, she stayed with the family.

When the family's younger child started preschool, they no longer needed the nanny fulltime, and she decided to take a few classes toward a degree in nursing. She planned to take three classes a week at a community college during the time the younger child was in school. She discussed this with the family, and they told her that they would have to think about it. A couple of months passed, and, since they had told her nothing, she thought they might have forgotten. They hadn't forgotten—they were not willing to let her take time to pursue a degree: "We can't 'allow' you to be away from the house that long. Besides, aren't you happy here?"

Delia stated that she was very happy, but that she had always wanted to fulfill her dream of being a nurse. Again the family told her they needed to think about it and nothing happened. Since the family had not consented to her taking the classes, she came to my agency seeking a position that would allow her to work in a family who would allow her to go to school in the mornings. She was still working with the family where she had been so long, and she decided to give them a two-week notice.

She was definitely marketable: she looked nice, spoke well, and had a valid U.S. driver's license. She cooked, cleaned, and she was great with children. Her previous references spoke highly of her. Since she was currently working for a family, I did not want to jeopardize her job. After two or three weeks, I found a family with twin girls looking for a live-in Monday-Friday. They were looking for someone with Delia's experience. She interviewed with the family and they wanted to hire her right away. She explained that she needed to give her current family a two-week notice.

Once the family called me and said they wanted to hire Delia, I called Delia to confirm that she wanted the new job. She said she did and that she would give her current employer notice. The following day I called the family where Delia worked and asked them a series of questions: "What type of person is Delia? Is she trustworthy? Does she get along well with the children? How are her cleaning skills? Why is she leaving?"

The mother told me that Delia was trustworthy, but that her children thought Delia was "okay"—that she did not interact much with them. She told me that her cleaning skills were not that good, but that she was all right. When I asked why she had kept her in her employ for five years, she said she did want to keep changing nannies.

As an agent, these answers left me between a rock and a hard place. Delia had told me that the family thought a great deal of her; the family had said that she was just "all right." As an agent, my job was to figure out who was telling the truth. I also had to tell the new family what her current family had said. Before I did, I called Delia to let her know that her reference was "okay." Of course, I did not repeat exactly what the employer had said. When the family that wanted to hire her asked me what the current employer had said, I told them, but I explained the entire story—Delia's side as well.

Her other references were fabulous, and I explained to the new family that they would also need to speak to Delia's employers themselves. After they did so, they decided that her present family just did not want her to leave. This interpretation was confirmed when they decided to "allow" her to take classes and begged her to stay.

Scenario 2:
Taking Advantage of a Caregiver

I had a client who had three daughters. The client was a single mother and a physician, and she needed reliable childcare. It was important to her that the nanny/housekeeper work Tuesday through Saturday because, like many single parents, she needed the caregiver to provide childcare over the weekend. The nanny arrived each Monday evening and left on Saturday evening. Sometimes the caregiver left first thing Sunday morning.

Staying until Sunday began to be routine; at first the client allowed the nanny to leave anytime Sunday morning, but soon the departure time turned into Sunday at noon. Additionally, the client rarely came home in the evenings; instead, she spent the night with her boyfriend. Consequently, it became the caregiver's sole responsibility to cook dinner, give the children baths, help them with their homework, and put them to bed. In essence, she was fully responsible for parenting three children of 6, 8, and 11. The client called in each evening to see how the children were doing.

When the nanny realized how routinely and how much she was being held responsible for, she called the agency. We had to explain to the client that she must come home in the evening to be with her children. The client was very upset, because she felt that the live-in was supposed to be there for her children. The client did not understand that *she* needed to raise her children—not the nanny. Certainly, the amount of care the client assumed the nanny would put in was far more than that outlined in the nanny's job description. After the agency intervened, the client realized that she was taking advantage of the nanny and started coming home each evening to be with her children.

Scenario 3:
The Attractive Blonde

Once I had a client who wanted a young nanny, someone in her early twenties who could be like a big sister to her seven-year-old twin daughters. She was looking for someone who could swim, play board games, take the children on outings, and do homework with them. She did not want an au pair. She wanted a nanny who would live in Monday through Friday.

Often nannies are out of state or even out of the country when they are hired, and clients do not meet them in person until they actually start working. They may have seen a photo during the interviewing process. In this case, I had interviewed the young woman who was to be their nanny. She was a Swedish girl who was working in Seattle, Washington. The family interviewed her by telephone and liked her immediately.

Two weeks later, the family sent for her to fly out for a face-to-face interview. The client later described the moment this way:

> When I opened the door, I saw a beautiful, tall, leggy blonde, Swedish girl. Once she sat down, I interviewed her, and she was lovely. She is everything we are looking for and more, but when my husband came home and entered the family room, his mouth dropped. Looking at him, I knew I could not have this beautiful young Swedish lady in my home.

The client called the agency and asked me to "Please find someone who is less attractive. I don't want any problems with the nanny and my husband." The agency found someone whom she felt was just as qualified and not quite so stunning to take over the role of big sister to the little girls.

Scenario 4:
The Dishonest Client

I had a client who was looking for a live-out nanny to work part-time three days a week. I had interviewed a 23-year-old who lived in the area. I called the young lady, Valerie, and she was very interested in the position. I called the clients back and told them I had some paperwork for them to fill out. I gave the family the phone number so they could set up an interview to meet with Valerie.

Once the interview took place, the family interviewed a few others through other agencies just to make some comparisons, which is good. The family told me that they had decided to hire someone else.

After two weeks of interviewing, the client stated that a friend of hers knew someone who was looking for a job and that they had interviewed her and hired her. The sequence of events struck me as suspicious: they really liked Valerie and they had been looking for some time; after they had interviewed Valerie, suddenly a friend found someone for them. Valerie, a nanny looking for a job, simultaneously stated that she had decided to go back to school full time.

I decided to look into this. I called an investigator who is a retired police officer who runs a private investigating business. We called the house during the hours the nanny would be working. When Valerie answered, I hung up. The investigator and I drove over and waited. Since I had interviewed the applicant, she knew what I looked like. I sat in the back of the truck with tinted windows, hidden, but I could see through the front windshield. At the time the nanny should be arriving for work, I saw a young, blond girl walking toward the house. We then knocked on the client's door, and Valerie opened it. The investigator immediately took pictures. I called the home, and the husband answered. I explained to him that his new nanny had been placed through my agency and that his wife had denied hiring her. The gentlemen said he would call back after he spoke to his wife. He did call back and said that his wife had hired Valerie through a friend who knew her and that they owed the agency nothing.

Prior to Valerie's being placed, I had had her fill out an affidavit, and that turned out to have been a fortunate act. I brought a civil suit against the client. Knowing that I had evidence to prove they were lying, the client did not want to go in front of a judge, and they decided to pay the agency fee. After that, I developed a pre-contract agreement.

Scenario 5:
Separated or Divorced Parents

I once placed a nanny with a single dad who had custody of his five daughters; they were between the ages of 4 and 13. The parents were in a major custody battle. When the mother called to talk to her daughters, she befriended the nanny. She began asking the nanny things about the father's girlfriend or what time he usually got home. What began as an isolated incident spiraled out of control. When the couple ended up in court, the husband had the nanny subpoenaed to appear in court, because the children had told him that the nanny had talked with their mom. He did not ask the nanny anything; he just had her subpoenaed. She told him that she knew nothing and gave her two-week notice and left. Parents need to remember not to make their problems, their caregiver's problems.

When hiring a caregiver, be mindful that this person is in your home fulfilling the valuable role of caring for your loved one(s).

Once a client and caregiver are properly matched, the household runs well. This smooth arrangement depends on your treating the caregiver with respect. This relationship, like so many others, will profit from remembering and practicing the "golden rule": "Do unto others as you would have them do unto you."

www.ingramcontent.com/pod-product-compliance
Lightning Source LLC
Chambersburg PA
CBHW022112170526
45157CB00004B/1594